High Blood Pressure

Vernon Coleman

What the papers say about Vernon Coleman and his books:

'Perhaps the best known health writer for the general public in the world today' - The Therapist

'The man is a national treasure' - What Doctors Don't Tell You

'Vernon Coleman writes brilliant books' - The Good Book Guide

'The revered guru of medicine' - Nursing Times

'A literary genius' - HSL Newsletter

'He's the Lone Ranger, Robin Hood and the Equalizer rolled into one' - Glasgow Evening Times

'Britain's leading health care campaigner' - The Sun

'Britain's leading medical author' - The Daily Star

'Brilliant' - The People

'Dr Vernon Coleman is one of our most enlightened, trenchant and sensible dispensers of medical advice' - The Observer

'The patient's champion' - Birmingham Post

'The medical expert you can't ignore' - Sunday Independent

'The most influential medical writer in Britain. There can be little doubt that Vernon Coleman is the people's doctor' - Devon Life

'The doctor who dares to speak his mind' - Oxford Mail

'Man with a mission' - Morning News

'Dr Coleman is more illuminating than the proverbial lady with the lamp' - Company Magazine

'Refreshingly sensible' - Spectator

'Dr Coleman gains in stature with successive books' - Coventry Evening Telegraph

'He writes lucidly and wittily' - Good Housekeeping

'The patient's champion. The doctor with the common touch' - Birmingham Post

'Clear and helpful' - The Guardian

'Vernon Coleman is a leading medical authority and known to millions through his writing, broadcasting and best selling books' - Womans Own

'His message is important' - The Economist

'It's impossible not to be impressed' - Western Daily Press

'A persuasive writer whose arguments, based on research and experience, are sound' - Nursing Standard

'His book Bodypower' is one of the most sensible treatises on personal survival that has ever been published' - Yorkshire Evening Post

'Dr Coleman is crusading for a more complete awareness of what is good and bad for our bodies. In the course of that he has made many friends and some powerful enemies' - Western Morning News

'His advice is optimistic and enthusiastic' - British Medical Journal

'The calmest voice of reason comes from Dr Vernon Coleman' - The Observer

'A godsend' - Daily Telegraph

A small selection from thousands of readers' letters:

'I admire your forthright and refreshingly honest way of expressing your views and opinions...bless you for being a light in the eternal darkness' - B.O.

'If only more people in the medical profession and this government were like you it would be a much nicer world' - G.W.

'My deep appreciation for your great courage and integrity over the years' - J.T.

'Truly, truly, I greatly admire the work you have done for both animals and man. I think you are wonderful and I wish I had but half your mind power and courage' - A.P.

'I admire your direct approach and philosophy in respect of general health, especially sexual health, environmental and animal issues' A.W.

'It's lovely to have someone who cares about people as you do. You tell us such a lot of things that we are afraid to ask our own doctors' K.C.

'I would like to thank you for telling us the truth' - R.K.

'I feel I must write and congratulate you ... your no-nonsense attitude, teamed with plain common sense makes a refreshing change. Please keep up the good work' - L.B.

'Thanks over and over again - good health always to you as you are fighting for a good cause in life - for the sick' - E.H.

'I only wish to God that we had a few such as your good self in Parliament, then maybe our standard of life would possibly be better' - H.H.

'I must admit that initially I thought that some of your ideas were extreme, but sadly I must concede that I was wrong' - C.D.

'I greatly admire your no nonsense approach to things and your acting as champion of the people' - L.A.

'I have now read and studied all your excellent books and have enjoyed and benefited from them immensely' - B.B.

'May I say that I think you have done a real service to all those who have the sense and patience to study your books' - B.A.

BOOKS BY VERNON COLEMAN

The Medicine Men (1975)
Paper Doctors (1976)
Everything You Want To Know About Ageing (1976)
Stress Control (1978)
The Home Pharmacy (1980)
Aspirin or Ambulance (1980)
Face Values (1981)
Guilt (1982)
The Good Medicine Guide (1982)
Stress And Your Stomach (1983)
Bodypower (1983)
An A to Z Of Women's Problems (1984)
Bodysense (1984)
Taking Care Of Your Skin (1984)
Life Without Tranquillisers (1985)
High Blood Pressure (1985)
Diabetes (1985)
Arthritis (1985)
Eczema and Dermatitis (1985)
The Story Of Medicine (1985)
Natural Pain Control (1986)
Mindpower (1986)
Addicts and Addictions (1986)
Dr Vernon Coleman's Guide To Alternative Medicine (1988)
Stress Management Techniques (1988)
Overcoming Stress (1988)
Know Yourself (1988)
The Health Scandal (1988)
The 20 Minute Health Check (1989)
Sex For Everyone (1989)
Mind Over Body (1989)
Eat Green Lose Weight (1990)
Toxic Stress (1991)

Why Animal Experiments Must Stop (1991)
The Drugs Myth (1992)
Why Doctors Do More Harm Than Good (1993)
Stress and Relaxation (1993)
Complete Guide to Sex (1993)
How to Conquer Backache (1993)
How to Conquer Arthritis (1993)
Betrayal of Trust (1994)
Know Your Drugs (1994)
Food for Thought (1994)
The Traditional Home Doctor (1994)
I Hope Your Penis Shrivels Up (1994)
People Watching (1995)
Relief from IBS (1995)
The Parent's Handbook (1995)
Oral Sex: Bad Taste And Hard To Swallow (1995)
Why Is Pubic Hair Curly? (1995)
Men in Dresses (1996)
Power over Cancer (1996)
Crossdressing (1996)
How You Can Get The Best Out Of Alternative Medicine (1996)
How You Can Get The Best Out Of Prescription Drugs (1996)
How to Stop Your Doctor Killing You (1996)
How to Overcome Toxic Stress (1996 rev)

novels
The Village Cricket Tour (1990)
The Bilbury Chronicles (1992)
Bilbury Grange (1993)
Mrs Caldicot's Cabbage War (1993)
The Man Who Inherited a Golf Course (1993)
Bilbury Revels (1994)
Deadline (1994)
Bilbury Country (1996)

short stories
Bilbury Pie (1995)

on cricket
Thomas Winsden's Cricketing Almanack (1983)
Diary Of A Cricket Lover (1984)

as Edward Vernon
Practice Makes Perfect (1977)
Practise What You Preach (1978)
Getting Into Practice (1979)
Aphrodisiacs - An Owners Manual (1983)
Aphrodisiacs - An Owners Manual (Turbo Edition) (1984)
The Complete Guide To Life (1984)

as Marc Charbonnier
Tunnel (novel 1980)

with Dr Alan C Turin
No More Headaches (1981)

with Alice
Alice's Diary (1989)
Alice's Adventures (1992)

High Blood Pressure

Vernon Coleman

European Medical Journal

Published in 1996 by the European Medical Journal, Publishing House.
Trinity Place, Barnstaple, Devon EX32 9HJ, England

Much of this book first appeared under the title 'Everything You Need To
Know About High Blood Pressure' in the series 'Dr Vernon Coleman's
Healthbooks for all the family', published by Severn House in 1985. This
edition first published in the United Kingdom by European Medical Journal
Books 1996.

Reprinted 1998 (twice), 1999 (twice)

ISBN: 1 898947 79 1

DEDICATION
To Tom and in the memory of Alice, Dick, Harry and Timmy

A catalogue record for this book is available from the British Library.

Printed and bound by: J.W. Arrowsmith Ltd., Bristol

NOTE 1

This book is not intended as an alternative to personal, professional medical advice. The reader should consult a physician in all matters relating to health, and particularly in respect of any symptoms which may require diagnosis or medical attention. While the advice and information in this book are believed to be accurate at the time of going to press, neither the author nor the publisher can accept any legal responsibility or liability for any errors or omission that may be made.

NOTE 2

You must consult your doctor before changing your diet or beginning any exercise programme. Following the advice in this book could have a dramatic effect on your blood pressure. If you learn to relax, cut out fats and lose weight, for example, there is a very good chance that your blood pressure will come down noticeably and your need for medication may change. It is, therefore, extremely important that before you follow the advice in this book and make any changes to your lifestyle you should tell your doctor exactly what you plan to do. You will need to visit him regularly so that he can check your blood pressure and find out whether or not your need for medication has altered.

CONTENTS

It is estimated that up to twenty per cent of the world's population have high blood pressure.
Only half of those know it.
Only half of those are being treated.
Only half of those are being treated effectively.

What is high blood pressure?

In order to survive and to thrive, the tissues and organs of the human body need regular supplies of fresh blood. It is blood that brings the oxygen and other essential foodstuffs without which the tissues would die, and it is blood that carries away the many waste products that are made. To travel around the body, through a complicated network of arteries, veins and capillaries, blood has to be kept under pressure. It is, of course, the heart which maintains that pressure, and it does this by regular, rhythmic pumping.

Under normal circumstances several factors affect the pressure at which blood travels around the body. First, there is the heart pump itself. If it is beating unusually rapidly or with exceptional force then that will obviously increase the pressure on the blood. Second, there is there is the size of the blood vessels, and in particular the muscular-walled arteries. If the bore of an artery has been narrowed then obviously the blood will have to be put under greater pressure for it to travel through the artery. Third, there is the amount of blood in the body. If the amount of blood increases for some reason then the pressure will rise: if the amount of blood falls then the pressure will fall.

Under normal circumstances blood pressure varies considerably. If, for example, you are being chased by a mugger then your body, recognising that your tissues need larger amounts of oxygen to cope with the crisis, will raise your blood pressure. This temporary variation will help you to stay alive. Once you have escaped from the mugger your blood pressure will go back to normal. Such a temporary change in blood pressure is acceptable and useful. It can, quite literally, help save your life.

Unfortunately, blood pressure sometimes goes up and stays up. And that can cause all sorts of problems. The tissues and organs around the body will be subjected to excessive pressures and there is a real risk that they will be damaged. If left unchecked, a persistent rise in blood pressure can kill. It is, for example, a major cause of heart disease and strokes. High blood pressure may not be an exciting, fashionable or dramatic disease and it may not attract much attention in the press or on television but it is one of the major causes of death in the world.

This book is designed to tell you everything you need to know about the causes of high blood pressure and about techniques which may help bring your blood pressure down. For, make no mistake about it, high blood pressure can in almost all cases, be treated both safely and effectively. And, most important of all it can, in many cases, be controlled partly or even completely without the use of drugs or other outside aids. When, in the 1970s, I first pointed out that high blood pressure could be brought down - and the need for medication reduced - I was attacked quite viciously by some in the medical profession who felt that the only way to treat high blood pressure was with the aid of drugs. I believe that today most doctors would agree with me that lifestyle changes are a vital part of good blood pressure control.

PART ONE

Fact-file on high blood pressure

What are the symptoms?

Most people who have high blood pressure have absolutely no symptoms at all. That is why high blood pressure is sometimes known as the 'silent killer'.

The only symptom that is reported with any regularity is a headache, usually at the back of the head and most often said to be worst in the mornings. Apart from that (and even the significance of the headache is disputed by some physicians) the only other symptoms sometimes experienced are dizziness and tiredness.

Individuals who have had persistent high blood pressure for some time will have symptoms produced not by their high blood pressure but by a problem or disease caused by the raised blood pressure. So, for example, patients may develop the sort of chest pains or breathlessness suggestive of heart disease. Occasionally, patients with high blood pressure may have strokes and may develop paralysis.

It is because high blood pressure is often quite symptomless that it is particularly important for it to be detected as early as possible by screening and routine check-ups. In this way it can be dealt with before any damage is done to the body.

How blood pressure is measured

The instrument used for measuring blood pressure is called a sphygmomanometer. When having your blood pressure taken you will normally be asked to sit down or lie down and relax as much as you possibly can. (Research has shown that when a doctor in a white coat approaches a patient the patient's blood pressure will usually rise.)

Once you are properly relaxed a rubber bag in a cloth sleeve will be wrapped around your upper arm and a rubber tube from that attached to the sphygmomanometer itself. (There are mercury, aneroid and electrical machines available, by the way, but the nature of the machine does not really affect the way the reading is measured.) As air is pumped into the bag the pressure inside the rubber bag is measured.

Then, releasing air from the bag, the person taking your blood pressure will place a stethoscope over the main artery in your arm so that he can measure the pressure under which blood is travelling around your body. Systolic pressure is the point at which he first hears blood managing to force itself through the flattened artery. The second, the diastolic pressure, is the point at which the sound fades away, eventually to disappear entirely.

There is no such thing as 'average' blood pressure since readings vary with age. It is also known that different doctors and nurses, taking the same individual's blood pressure will come up with different readings. So it is important that the same person takes your blood pressure every time.

When your doctor checks your blood pressure he may also look into your eyes. He does this because the retina at the back of the eye is covered with many small arteries. This is, indeed, the only place where the condition of the arteries can be inspected. Your doctor may also check your urine (to see if there are any signs of kidney damage) and take a chest X-ray and electrocardiograph to see if your heart has been affected by your blood pressure.

Malignant or essential

There are two main types of high blood pressure: malignant and essential.

Malignant, much the rarer of the two and also known as accelerated or secondary, is usually much the higher and more threatening of the two. There are usually signs of some damage to the body's organs. This type of high blood pressure usually develops fairly rapidly and can kill. Although it may be difficult to isolate the specific cause of malignant high blood pressure the basic problem often involves the kidneys where some physiological or pathological malfunction results in the over production of a substance called renin. The over production of renin results in a retention of salt, a rise in the volume of blood and a constriction of blood vessel walls.

In about ninety-five per cent of cases of high blood pressure it will be of the essential type. In these cases there will be no specific identifiable cause.

It is malignant high blood pressure that usually needs hospital attention. Essential high blood pressure will usually be treated without any need for an appointment with a hospital specialist.

Does high blood pressure affect life expectancy?

Your body can cope with temporary increases in blood pressure very well. A permanent increase in blood pressure can, however, cause severe damage and reduce your life expectancy.

At the age of thirty-five a man with a blood pressure of 120/80 can expect to live another forty-one and a half years. At the same age a man with a blood pressure of 150/100 can expect to live another twenty-five years.

(These two figures represent the readings obtained when measuring the highest and lowest pressures at which blood is being pumped around your body. The highest figure is the 'systolic', the lowest the 'diastolic'.)

At the age of forty-five a man with a blood pressure of 120/80 can expect to live another thirty-two years. A man of the same age with a blood pressure of 150/100 can expect to live another twenty and a half years.

At the age of fifty-five a man with a blood pressure of 120/80 can expect to live another twenty-three and a half years. A man of the same age with a blood pressure of 150/100 can expect to live another seventeen and a half years.

For women the figures are similar although slightly less dramatic.

At the age of forty-five a woman with a blood pressure of 120/80 can expect to live another thirty-seven years. A woman of the same age with a blood pressure of 150/100 can expect to live another twenty-eight and a half years.

A good many other factors affect life expectancy but I feel that these figures do show just how dangerous high blood pressure can be. It is, it seems to me, quite clear that anyone who has a raised blood pressure should, with their doctor's help and approval, do everything they can do to bring their blood pressure down and under control. The improvement in life expectancy can be quite significant.

How high blood pressure will affect your life

Until your blood pressure is under control you should take care not to get too excited, not to expose yourself to extraordinary stresses (changing job or moving house) and not to start to take violent exercise. Any one of these circumstances will send your blood pressure up. Obviously, if your pressure is already high the additional rise could prove dangerous.

Sex is naturally one area that worries patients with high blood pressure (and, inevitably, it worries their partners too).

It is, of course, perfectly true that energetic sexual activity puts an extra strain on the circulatory system. In practice major problems during intercourse are relatively rare. But that does not mean that the risk should not be acknowledged or taken seriously.

When patients do collapse, develop heart disease or have a stroke during intercourse it is usually because the circumstances are in some way exceptional. So, for example, the older man who eats too much, drinks too much and then tries to impress a young girl with his virility will be at risk. Patients having extra-marital sex (where the feelings of guilt are greater than usual) are particularly at risk.

In general, my advice to patients with high blood pressure has to be that they should enjoy a normal, healthy sex life but remember that until their blood pressure is under control they may need to be a trifle cautious and perhaps even restrained in their love making. Avoid drinking too much or eating a lot before sex and avoid adultery and sexual practices likely to lead to extra stress.

Incidentally, some drugs used to control high blood pressure may produce temporary problems - such as impotence. If this happens report to your doctor straight away.

Apart from encouraging patients to adapt their lifestyle according to the blood pressure control programme, the only other advice I would give is that they should try to get up slowly when they have been in bed or in an armchair (changing position changes the blood pressure and can produce sudden dizziness) and take warm, rather than hot, baths since immersion in hot water can cause a sudden change in blood pressure.

What causes high blood pressure?

Only in a relatively small number of instances of high blood pressure can specific, identifiable causes be found. There may, for example, be an inherited anatomical problem offering some exceptional obstruction to the flow of blood around the body thereby affecting the overall blood pressure. The adrenal glands which have the job of producing the sort of hormones which stimulate a response to stress and danger may be diseased in some way and may, in consequence, over produce their vital hormones - with the result that the body reacts as though it were constantly under pressure. If there are too many red cells in the blood because of some internal production problem then the blood will be too thick and the blood pressure will rise accordingly because pushing thick, cell-heavy blood around the body requires extra pressure.

In the ninety-five per cent of cases where high blood pressure develops without there being any logical physiological or pathological explanation there are very often identifiable factors which link various groups of patients together. Whether or not these factors are themselves linked in some way is still a mystery.

On the pages which follow I shall deal with the commonest and most important factors known to cause a rise in blood pressure. If you are a sufferer it is important to read through these pages carefully and see if you can spot which causes are likely to be responsible for your particular case. Once you have identified the factors which you think could be responsible for your high blood pressure you should turn to the appropriate advice. By changing your lifestyle in some way it will very probably be possible for you to bring your blood pressure down to normal again. A high proportion of those patients who have high blood pressure for which there is no straightforward explanation will be able to reduce it to normal simply by identifying causative factors and then dealing with those factors in the ways suggested. And even in those patients where the blood pressure cannot be controlled by dealing with causative factors it will almost always be possible to obtain some improvement by following the advice that I have listed.

Understand what is causing your high blood pressure and you stand a very good chance of being able to control it without drugs of any kind.

Genetics

No one really knows just how high blood pressure is transmitted from generation to generation but there is now little doubt that it is quite possible to inherit a tendency to develop high blood pressure. If your father or mother had high blood pressure then you have a greater than average chance of developing it yourself.

If both your parents had high blood pressure then, it seems, your chances of developing it are even greater.

All this means that if you do not have high blood pressure yourself but you have close relatives who have high blood pressure (parents and brother and sisters) then you should have your blood pressure checked once a year as a routine precaution. Similarly, if you yourself have high blood pressure then you should encourage your own close relatives to visit their doctor once a year for a check-up.

Incidentally, according to the latest information available it seems most likely that when an individual inherits high blood pressure it is because he has inherited either a susceptibility to salt or a sensitivity to stress. So when high blood pressure runs in a family it might be sensible for all concerned to take particular note of these two factors.

What is perhaps even more remarkable is that we probably acquire our adult blood pressure relatively early in our lives. It seems that if we are destined to end up with high blood pressure as adults we will have had a higher than average blood pressure throughout childhood. By the time we reach eighteen our future destiny is well and truly settled.

All this suggests that since high blood pressure is a major cause of death and disease in the Western world, and is now recognised to have reached epidemic proportions in many parts, we ought to be screening school children for early signs of a blood pressure problem. It would be relatively simple for children to be screened in their mid-teens and would, in financial terms, prove a sound proposition since the long term saving on medical manpower and materials would be massive.

Personality

During recent years, researchers all around the world have been trying to find out whether or not there is any fundamental difference between the sorts of individuals who develop peptic ulcers, the types who get cancer and the sorts who end up with high blood pressure.

It is, after all, relatively rare for one individual to suffer from more than one major disease. So it is reasonable to assume that some physical or mental characteristic must decide which particular problem will affect which individual.

The evidence which has been accumulated so far suggests that the most important factor is personality.

Psychologists and psychiatrists and trained observers of all kinds now claim that it is possible to predict just what sort of person ends up with which type of disease. This information is valuable for two reasons.

First, because we know now what sort of people get asthma, for example, we can pick out those individuals, and help them reduce their risks of exacerbating that particular problem. It is not possible to change anyone's personality, of course, but it is often possible to adapt or alter one's attitudes, habits and behavioural patterns. And, of course, it is also possible to reduce other risk factors. So, for example, with someone whose personality marks him as an asthma risk avoiding cigarettes is a priority.

Second, once an individual has been diagnosed as suffering from a particular ailment (such as high blood pressure) it is often possible to help that individual get better by teaching him how to adapt his approach to life. If your personality, attitude and approach to life have caused a specific problem then by altering them you can often solve or lessen it.

The following list of traits is not intended to provide a pen picture of all high blood pressure patients, of course. It is unlikely that any one patient will fit perfectly into the pattern that has been recorded (and, indeed, it is possible for an individual who has none of these personality traits to develop high blood pressure for there are, of course, factors other than personality involved).

However, if you are a sufferer look through this list and see whether or not you recognise yourself or your own behavioural pattern.

• People who are prone to high blood pressure, are, like people who are prone to heart disease, often quite aggressive and competitive. If you are competitive you are probably very ambitious as well. That in itself is not necessarily dangerous, of course. But if you find it difficult to relax and to stop pushing yourself to succeed then you probably do have a problem which needs dealing with.

• You may well need to do everything quickly. High blood pressure sufferers tend to be impatient and to get irritable when they are slowed down or frustrated by others. So, for example, people who get high blood pressure tend to get very irritated when they find themselves in traffic jams - and that does not do their blood pressure any good at all.

• If it is your personality that has made you liable to high blood pressure then you probably find it difficult to relax. You may even feel guilty if you sit down and do nothing. You may feel the urge to keep moving all the time and to be doing something 'useful' every minute of the day. You probably hate holidays by the sea where people lie around all day doing nothing. And you probably feel more comfortable if you have got some work with you or if you can hurry from cathedral to museum and back again.

• You are almost certainly extra sensitive to stress. For years many people have been bewildered by the fact that some individuals seem to cope extremely well with enormous amounts of stress and others crack up when the stress levels are still modest. The simple truth is, of course, that we all respond differently to stress and we all have different stress thresholds.

• It is not the amount of stress that we are subjected to which causes the problems, so much as our ability to cope with it. If you have a fairly low stress threshold you are likely to suffer even if your job and home life are relatively peaceful. Just missing a bus or finding that a button has come off a shirt will be enough to cause you worry and anxiety. If you have a high stress threshold you will be able to cope perfectly well with circumstances which might put someone else in hospital.

• It is not particularly comforting to know this but if you are the sort of individual who suffers badly from stress and pressure then you can at least console yourself with the thought that if you ever get stranded on a desert island or stuck in the jungle you would probably survive much better than someone who does not respond to stressful situations. If you are the sort who suffers when under stress then you probably have good reflexes, you probably wake up quickly if a sudden noise breaks the stillness of the night and your body probably reacts fairly rapidly to physical danger. All those responses would make you more capable of coping in an environment where physical danger was the main threat. Unfortunately, those responses make you ill-equipped to cope with twentieth-century living. However, do not despair. Even if you do over-react to stress there is still much that you can do to protect yourself.

• You probably become angry fairly easily and you may well shout when you are cross. You probably over-react sometimes and find yourself getting a little out of control. In extreme cases high blood pressure sufferers have hair-trigger tempers.

• A large percentage of the people who get high blood pressure repress their negative emotions. So, for example, when you are upset or sad you may refuse to cry, and refuse to let people see just how upset you really are. This sort of attitude is particularly prevalent among males who will almost certainly have been taught as boys to suppress emotions.

• You probably carry more guilt than is your fair share. Individuals who suffer from blood pressure problems tend to be happy to take the blame when things go wrong, they tend to worry about what other people think and they tend to be unselfish.

• You are almost certainly a worrier. You probably worry about just about anything that comes your way. You worry about whether or not you are going to have enough money (even if you have enough for your needs); you worry about the weather; you worry about whether you are doing a good job; you worry about whether other people are happy. And, of course, you worry about having high blood pressure.

Remember, of course, that not all blood pressure sufferers will exhibit all these personality traits. But look through the list and see just which ones apply to you. Then you can find out how to adapt your personality so that you can cope more effectively with life. And do remember too, by the way, that I am not suggesting that any of the traits mentioned here are bad ones. Some of these are traits which make you a good reliable, honest individual. These are not traits which need to be eradicated. But when problems like high blood pressure ensue they will need controlling a little.

Stress

I firmly believe that one of the most important (if not the most important) reasons for the apparent epidemic of high blood pressure these days is the fearful increase in the amount of stress that we all have to cope with.

That may sound a strange argument. After all, most of us these days have plenty of food to eat. We have somewhere warm and dry to sleep every night and we do not have to worry too much about being attacked or eaten by wild animals. Compared to our ancestors we would, on the surface, appear to have an easy life. You would not really think that we were more likely to suffer from stress-induced diseases than our ancestors, would you?

I think the reason why we do suffer so much, and why blood pressure is now one of the commonest and most dangerous disorders in the Western world, is that our bodies were not designed for the sort of stress we have to endure these days. We were designed for an instant world.

If you turn a corner and come face to face with a man-eating tiger then your body will react remarkably well to that instant threat.

Your heart will beat faster in order to ensure that as much blood as possible reaches your muscles (this will ensure that plenty of oxygen reaches the tissues which need it to help you cope with the emergency); acid will pour into your stomach (this ensures that any food there is converted into usable energy and reaches your blood stream just as speedily as possible); and your muscles will tense (to ensure that you are well prepared for fighting the tiger, running away from it or climbing up the nearest tree).

Those are just three of the natural, physical responses your body makes to stress. There are many more.

Now, in the sort of world our ancestors lived in a few thousand years ago that sort of response would have helped to keep them alive. If you could run, fight and climb then you had a good chance of surviving. Those traits were handed down from father to son simply because the individuals who were not very good at running, jumping, climbing and fighting (in other words the individuals whose muscles did not tense and whose hearts did not beat faster) were all eaten by marauding, man-eating tigers.

Unfortunately, in our modern world those natural, automatic responses are not always appropriate. Indeed, they are sometimes a hindrance rather than a help.

The trouble is that we have changed our world far quicker than our bodies have been able to evolve. Revolutionary changes in navigation, medicine, science, military tactics, agriculture, industry and so on have changed the world a great deal. These days there are not many man-eating tigers wandering around. And most of our threats and problems cannot be solved by physical action.

The simple truth is that we have changed our world too much. Our bodies have just not been able to cope. Today we respond to danger in exactly the same way that our ancestors responded thousands of years ago. But today the dangers and threats are different.

These days we do not have to worry about being eaten: we have to worry about paying our bills, keeping our jobs, coping with inflation, fighting off court summonses, policemen and traffic wardens, and dealing with the million-and-one administrators and bureaucrats who impinge on our lives.

Our bodies respond to these modern threats in exactly the same way that they would have responded to a man-eating tiger: the heart beats faster, the blood pressure goes up, the muscles become tense and so on.

Unfortunately, these responses, although perfectly natural, are quite inappropriate.

If you have bills to pay, a job to find or a parking ticket to pay, those natural, physiological responses will not help you at all. Increased muscle tension and a higher blood pressure will help you run or fight. But those responses will not help you deal with piles of paperwork or officious administrators.

Worse still, because our modern problems tend to go on and on for long periods, the natural stress response remains switched on and our muscles stay tense and our hearts continue to beat faster for months or even years. The muscles remain tense, the heart beats faster and the blood pressure stays high for far too long - with the result that your body actually damages itself. What was intended as a protective response has become a damaging one.

Understand all this and it becomes easy to see why stress is one of the main causes of high blood pressure. It is also to easy to see just why it is important for anyone who suffers from high blood pressure to learn how to cope with stress.

Is stress affecting your blood pressure?

Some people are much more susceptible to stress than others. While one individual will be able to cope perfectly well with an apparently endless series of major crises, another will be sent into a state of panic at the thought of missing a train or the sight of a button coming off a shirt. Our stress thresholds vary enormously and so it is helpful to know just how vulnerable you are to stress. If you have a high stress threshold you will be able to cope with tremendous pressures - indeed you may even enjoy being under a good deal of pressure. If, on the other hand, you have a low stress threshold then you will need to minimise your exposure to stress if you want to keep your blood pressure under control.

To benefit from the quiz which follows you must answer all the questions - and answer them accurately.

1.   *Do you get physical symptoms such as headaches, indigestion, vomiting or diarrhoea before important appointments or meetings?*
     a)   always
     b)   never
     c)   sometimes

2.   *When you are anxious or excited, does your:*
     a)   pulse race and your heart pound?
     b)   your pulse increase a small amount?

c)   your pulse stay much the same as usual?

3.   *If you are concentrating hard on what you are doing and someone suddenly comes up behind you, do you:*
a)   jump a mile?
b)   respond involuntarily but quickly get control of your self?
c)   remain calm and unperturbed?

4.   *When you are frightened or anxious or upset, does your face:*
a)   stay much the same as usual?
b)   go a little pale?
c)   go quite white?

5.   *When you get upset or nervous, do you:*
a)   get butterflies in your stomach and sweat a good deal?
b)   get just one of those symptoms?
c)   get neither of them?

6.   *What is your reaction time like?*
a)   below average?
b)   average
c)   above average, very fast

7.   *Do you ever have difficulty in breathing when you are excited?*
a)   often
b)   occasionally
c)   never

8.   *When you become angry or furious, does your face:*
a)   stay the same as usual?
b)   redden a little?
c)   go bright red?

9.   *If you are waiting for an important phone call which does*
      not come, do you:
      a)   become a nervous wreck?
      b)   get a bit edgy?
      c)   remain quite calm?

10.   *If, when you are lying in bed at night, you are suddenly*
      woken by an unexpected noise, do you:
      a)   wake up quickly and completely?
      b)   take ages to wake up and realise what has happened?
      c)   wake up quickly but take a few seconds to realise ex-
            actly what has happened?

Now add up your score.

1	a3	b1	c2
2	a3	b2	c1
3	a3	b2	c1
4	a1	b2	c3
5	a3	b2	c1
6	a1	b2	c3
7	a3	b2	c1
8	a1	b2	c3
9	a3	b2	c1
10	a3	b1	c2

If you scored between 20 and 30 you are the sort of individual who
would survive well in a world where physical dangers posed a threat.
You would stand a good chance of surviving in the jungle, for example, where your fast reactions would help you look after yourself.
On the other hand, you are not, I am afraid, well suited for our
modern world. And your high blood pressure is likely to have been
caused or made worse by your response to stress. You will probably be able to reduce your blood pressure by learning to avoid
excessive stress, and by learning to increase your capacity to cope

with stressful situations.

If you scored between 13 and 19 then you are very much in the middle range, between the two extremes. You would probably still benefit from learning how to control your responses to stress.

If you scored 12 or less you would probably not last long in the jungle or in any sort of environment where physical threats are common. But you are fairly well adapted to life in the modern world. It is unlikely that your high blood pressure has been caused by your responses to stress.

Weight

According to one major study, if you are twenty per cent or more overweight your chances of developing high blood pressure are increased ten-fold. Equally important, there is evidence to show that it is by increasing the blood pressure that extra, excess weight produces heart disease.

For those who are prepared to lose excess weight the news is very encouraging. It has been shown that substantial weight reduction is at least as effective as any of the popularly prescribed 'first choice' anti-hypertensive drugs.

In other words, if an overweight patient with high blood pressure can lose that excess weight then the chances are good that his or her blood pressure will return to normal.

Exactly why excess weight puts the blood pressure up is still something of a mystery but there are a couple of quite logical explanations available. First, it is perfectly possible that the blood pressure needs to go up for the very simple reason that there is more body to provide with fresh supplies of blood. If the pressure does not rise then the more distant parts of the body will not receive any blood. If you want to squirt water a long way out of a hose then you have to turn up the pressure. Second, it is also reasonable to assume that individuals who are overweight will have eaten too much salt (because they eat a lot of food) - and salt seems to be a common factor in exacerbating blood pressure problems in susceptible individuals.

Salt

It has been recognised for centuries that too much salt can cause damage. Even the Egyptian priests regarded it as a potential health hazard. The first scientists to argue that salt could cause harm were Ambard and Beaujard who, in 1904, published papers prescribing a link between salt consumption and high blood pressure. Despite this early start it was not until the 1940s that more clinical research work was published and the link between salt and hypertension firmly established. The problem then was that the recommended diet for hypertensives was, for many, simply too unpalatable. Patients who have symptom-free high blood pressure are notoriously (and understandably) reluctant to accept forms of treatment which are unpleasant. Trying to cut out all the foods that contain salt can result in a rather dull diet.

Until quite recently it was not just the difficulty of persuading people to stick to a salt-free diet that stopped doctors recommending such a solution for high blood pressure. Another problem was that, despite many research attempts, no one had managed to find out just why some people could eat lots of salt without it affecting their blood pressure while others seemed to suffer enormously if they ate modest amounts.

A year or two ago an explanation for this phenomenon was found. Those individuals whose blood pressure is adversely affected by salt are in some way genetically susceptible to it. They develop high blood pressure when they eat salt (and these days most of us living in the Western world eat too much salt - it just happens to play a fairly important part in the sort of diet we are used to) simply because they are extra sensitive to it and their bodies are unable to cope with the excesses.

If you suffer from high blood pressure then there must be a

risk that excess salt will be making your blood pressure worse. Cut down your consumption of salt and your blood pressure may fall.

Cholesterol and Fats

I believe that if you eat unlimited animal fats then you will run a much higher than average risk of having high blood pressure, a heart attack or a stroke.

The first link between fat intake and heart disease was noticed way back in the early 1950s. Since then much more evidence has been accumulated.

In my view anyone with raised blood pressure would be foolish not to cut down their consumption of animal fats.

Coffee and Tea

A number of reports have been published in recent years suggesting that caffeine may cause high blood pressure. I believe that sufferers would do well to cut down their consumption of drinks (for example, coffee, tea and cola drinks) which contain caffeine.

Skin Colour

Just why skin colour should affect blood pressure is still something of a mystery, but if you are black you are much more likely to suffer from high blood pressure than if you are white. And you are more likely to die from problems (such as stroke or heart disease) caused by your blood pressure.

Attempts to come up with explanations for this have produced a number of possible answers. It has been suggested, for example, that it is the stress of living in a hostile environment which produces the high blood pressure. Blacks, it is argued, are much more likely to have problems in achieving financial stability and they are more likely to be harassed by the police and by employers.

This theory is certainly substantiated by evidence which shows that when blacks migrate to urban areas where stress is greater they have a greater chance of developing hypertension.

Another quite logical explanation is that dietary factors are responsible. Many blacks live on a diet which contains much more salt, saturated fat and cholesterol than is healthy. Foods such as pork ribs, ham and salty bacon are all particularly rich in salt and fat.

Smoking

Individuals who have high blood pressure and who smoke are often recommended to give it up as soon as they possibly can. There are sound, clinical reasons for this. Although the statistics vary, of course, from area to area and from patient to patient there is sound evidence to show that if you have high blood pressure then you have a twice as normal chance of having a heart attack. If, however, you have high blood pressure and you smoke then your chances of having a heart attack are multiplied by four. There is also evidence which shows that if you smoke and you have high blood pressure your chances of having a stroke will be similarly increased.

Different doctors offer various explanations for these statistics. Some argue that smoking increases the blood pressure, others claim that smoking creates symptoms, such as nervousness, which in turn lead to higher blood pressure. Exactly what the mechanisms are is relatively unimportant, however. What is unarguable is that there is a relationship between smoking, high blood pressure, heart disease and strokes.

Also true, and far more encouraging, is the evidence which shows that if you manage to give up smoking then your chances of having a heart attack or a stroke will be dramatically reduced. There is, therefore, a very sound reason for people with high blood pressure to keep away from tobacco. (And that means keeping away from other people who smoke as well as not smoking!)

Noise

We are all more or less permanently surrounded by noise. The noise of cars, buses and lorries, the noise of machinery and office equipment and the noise of several million radio and television sets provides a background against which can be set the more spectacular noises of aircraft and road repairers.

All this noise undoubtedly has a harmful effect. It disturbs our ability to concentrate; it produces fatigue and bad temper and results in damaged hearing. It affects our ability to talk to each other and it increases our chances of having accidents. Because noise results in the tensing of muscles it can also produce headaches and high blood pressure. Research done with factory workers has shown, quite conclusively, that there is a real link between noise and the development of high blood pressure. Even more important, however, the research showed that when the workers were given ear muffs those individuals whose blood pressure had risen made a remarkable recovery.

The message is, therefore, quite simple. If you spend your days working in a noisy environment then it is important that you do what you can to shield yourself from it. Providing yourself with some protection may well help reduce your blood pressure. If your blood pressure is normal then keeping unwanted noises out may help keep it that way.

Pregnancy

About one in four women suffer from a raised blood pressure at some stage during their pregnancy. The raised blood pressure may be accompanied by a swelling of the hands and legs and by the presence of measurable amounts of protein in the urine.

It is partly in order to detect a rise in blood pressure that expectant mothers are instructed to visit their doctors regularly during the months prior to delivery.

The treatment for this type of high blood pressure varies but most women are advised to learn how to relax, to spend some time resting each day and to avoid the consumption of salt. Some women may need to take drugs to reduce their blood pressure.

Occasionally, when the blood pressure rises uncontrollably a woman may need to be taken into hospital to have her labour induced a little early. This is, however, relatively rare.

In most cases when the blood pressure has risen during pregnancy it will go back down again after the baby is delivered though it may recur during a future pregnancy.

Drugs

Although the contraceptive pill is probably the commonest and most widely known offender it is not the only drug likely to cause high blood pressure. There are a number of other drugs which can, in some patients, produce a noticeable and sometimes dangerous rise in pressure.

I would suggest that anyone who has high blood pressure and who takes medication (prescribed or bought over the counter) for any other condition should ask their doctor whether the medication could be responsible for making their blood pressure worse.

All women taking the contraceptive pill should have regular blood pressure checks done at intervals of six months. If a check-up shows that there has been a rise in the blood pressure then the obvious solution is to change to some other form of contraception. When the pill is stopped the blood pressure will usually return to normal within about three months.

Alcohol

A modest consumption of alcohol does not have any adverse effects on blood pressure. In fact, a small amount of alcohol each day may help keep the blood pressure down. When the consumption of alcohol becomes heavier, however, the pressure can be pushed up fairly considerably. And since alcohol is usually rich in calories, heavy drinking invariably also means an increase in weight - and that in turn has an additional deleterious effect on the blood pressure.

PART TWO

Doctors and Drugs:
medical treatments

The role of the general practitioner

Once you have been diagnosed as suffering from high blood pressure your general practitioner or family doctor will play an important part in your treatment.

Whether or not your high blood pressure is first identified by your family doctor, you should visit him as soon as possible to tell him exactly what has been found. If your high blood pressure was discovered during a routine insurance examination or at a medical examination for a job then the doctor who performed the tests will probably write to your own doctor anyway. He certainly should do so.

When confronted with patients who have raised blood pressure, some general practitioners begin treatment with drugs straight away. Indeed, there are many medical practitioners who firmly believe that all patients with high blood pressure will need to stay on drugs for the rest of their lives. Since most doctors get their information about diseases and drugs from drug companies, and since drug companies like selling products for years and years, it is hardly surprising that too few doctors are aware that blood pressure problems can be treated without drugs.

Whether or not your doctor suggests that you try reducing your blood pressure yourself there is nothing to stop you following my blood pressure control programme and trying to 'help' the drug treatment that has been prescribed. You must, of course, tell your doctor what you plan to do and ask for his permission and approval.

Once your high blood pressure has been diagnosed you should visit your doctor regularly so that he can keep a check on it. You should do this whether or not you are receiving any drug therapy and whether or not you are trying to reduce your blood pressure yourself.

To begin with I suggest that you visit the surgery once a week or once a fortnight. Obviously, however, you will need to be guided by your doctor as to when you should return to the surgery. In some instances the family doctor may want to see a patient every couple of days.

If your doctor gives you a prescription and tells you to return to the surgery in a couple of months time then I suggest you change your doctor. In order to have your blood pressure controlled effectively you will need to be seen regularly.

When your general practitioner checks your blood pressure at future visits he will be anxious to see just how well the treatments you have been trying are controlling your blood pressure. If, despite all your own efforts and despite the drugs that you have been prescribed, your blood pressure has not fallen your doctor will probably prescribe a more powerful product.

Just how often he will want to see you will, of course, depend on exactly how well the blood pressure is controlled. If it is controlled well then you may eventually need only attend every three or six months. I do not think that anyone receiving treatment for high blood pressure should go for more than six months without having a check-up.

Because high blood pressure is a common problem and because it can usually be controlled quite effectively by using drugs or by changing your lifestyle, few patients with blood pressure problems are referred to a hospital specialist. If, however, the blood pressure cannot easily be controlled or is uncomfortably high then your general practitioner will resort to this.

Since high blood pressure is a potentially hazardous condition you should never have to wait more than one week for an appointment if it has been decided that a specialist's opinion is necessary.

Getting the best out of your doctor

Far too many patients come out of a doctor's surgery and then remember that they have forgotten to tell him something that was important, or to ask something that they really needed to know.

There are many explanations for this, of course. First, most people worry about their health. That is perfectly natural, So, when they need to see a doctor they tend to be nervous and anxious. It is hardly surprising that they forget what they wanted to say. And, second, the advice that doctors give can be lengthy and involve such things as how to take tablets, when to come back to the surgery, what side effects to watch out for, and so on and so on.

I think that when you are going to see your doctor you should plan your visit carefully, and before going sit down for a few minutes and try to think of everything that you want to tell him - and everything you want to ask him. Then note it all down on a piece of paper.

You must, obviously, tell him about any symptoms you have. Tell him not just about the ones that seem important to you but of everything else you may have noticed too. Something that seems irrelevant to you may provide a vital clue.

On your first visit to the surgery tell him about any close relatives who also have high blood pressure, and be prepared to answer questions about your weight, your diet, your smoking habits and your daily exercise habits. If you have a past history of any disease then tell him about that too. Your doctor may have forgotten or the information may be 'lost' in your files. Your doctor will probably want to know something about your job because how you spend your day will have some effect on your blood pressure - so be prepared for questions about your work.

It is also wise to tell him about any pills, tablets or medicines you are already taking; whether they are products that have been prescribed or products that you have bought over the chemist's counter.

Remember too to jot down any specific questions that you want to ask. You may want to know whether you can carry on mountaineering, or whether you should temporarily retire from Grand Prix motor racing.

Write down all the questions you want answered. Obviously, if you go in to see your doctor clutching a huge three hundred page account of your medical history and you have hundreds of questions to ask then he is going to become a little impatient. But he will not mind at all if you go in with a few notes jotted down. Indeed, he will almost certainly appreciate the fact that you are trying to help him help you get better.

And write down the advice he gives you. If he gives you information about your pills make a note of what he tells you. Make a note about the dosage, about any possible side effects, about when to stop taking the pills, about whether or not you need to avoid any particular food or alcohol while on the drugs.

Make a careful note too about when you have got to go back to the surgery, about whether or not you need to see anyone at the hospital and, if you do need to see a specialist, the name of the doctor he is referring you to.

Doctors write down everything you tell them. And there is absolutely no reason at all why you should not write down everything the doctor tells you.

The role of the hospital specialist

Unless your blood pressure is unusually high or difficult to control you are unlikely to need to see a hospital specialist. Under some circumstances, however, you may have to.

So, for example, if your general practitioner cannot control your blood pressure with the drugs he is familiar with he may arrange an appointment with a specialist so that he can obtain some advice about other drugs to try. New products are coming onto the market every month and no general practitioner can possibly hope to keep up to date with all the latest products. Referring a patient to a hospital specialist for treatment advice is a sign of strength not weakness.

You are likely to need to go into hospital for treatment of high blood pressure under three separate sets of circumstances:

• If your doctor or your specialist suspect that there may be an underlying cause for your high blood pressure then they will probably take you into hospital for tests to be done. Some of the equipment used these days is extremely sophisticated and needs expert technicians if useful results are going to be obtained. You are also likely to need to go into hospital if your doctor finds that there is a cause for your high blood pressure and that the cause needs treatment (for example, a problem that needs a surgical operation).

• If your blood pressure is unusually high then your doctor may decide that it will be better to treat your blood pressure in hospital simply so that it will be possible to bring it under control more speedily. In hospital doctors can change your treatment hourly if they wish. They can also give treatments by injection instead of by mouth and most drugs work faster when passed straight into the tissues.

• If your blood pressure is difficult to control then you may need to go into hospital for a few days while different drugs are tried.

Always remember, however, that even if your blood pressure is high or difficult to control there will nearly always be a drug available which will control it. Once your blood pressure problem has been identified treatment is usually a matter of trial and error until a suitable therapeutic agent is found.

When does high blood pressure need treating with drugs?

If you asked this question of a hundred doctors you would probably receive a hundred different answers.

At one extreme there are many doctors who claim that a high proportion of patients with 'higher-than-average' blood pressure can be controlled by, changing their diet, losing weight and reducing their exposure to stress. This is a philosophy which I favour.

At the other extreme there are those doctors who believe that every patient with high blood pressure should receive drug treatment.

It has been said that patients who have a diastolic pressure below 90mm of mercury do not need treatment and that those patients who have a diastolic pressure between 90mm of mercury and 95mm of mercury need to have their blood pressure checked every three months but do not need drug therapy.

Those patients should, of course, be given advice about diet and stress control.

I think many doctors would agree that patients who have a diastolic pressure above 95mm of mercury should be started on drug treatment.

The evidence suggests that if you have high blood pressure and your doctor prescribes for you then you should, perhaps, ask whether or not your prescription is really necessary. You should also ensure that your blood pressure is checked regularly so that as soon as it falls your treatment can be stopped or at least adjusted. You must always tell your doctor if you intend to change your lifestyle - either by changing your diet, giving up smoking, taking up exercise or losing weight. Tell him exactly what you intend to do and ask for his approval, support and guidance.

Drugs for high blood pressure

There are scores of drugs available for the treatment of high blood pressure and to be perfectly honest I doubt if there are many doctors in practice who have ever even heard of all the available products. Many patients with high blood pressure need to keep taking drugs for months or even years - that means that there are huge potential profits to be won by companies which can market safe and effective drugs. It is hardly surprising, therefore, that most of the major international companies produce at least one drug designed for the treatment of high blood pressure.

Getting the best out of prescribed drugs

Drugs can be dangerous, it is true. But they can be extraordinarily useful. And, if drugs help bring your blood pressure down to normal then they can save your life. To get the best out of drugs, while at the same time minimising the risks you run, you need to know how to use drugs safely and effectively. Read through the following notes.

1. Always make sure that you find out as much as you can about the drugs you have been given. If your doctor does not tell you when your drugs need to be taken then ask him for the information - he may forget to put the advice on your prescription. The most important things you need to know are:

a) For how long the drug needs to be taken. Usually, drugs given for high blood pressure need to be taken continuously, at least until your blood pressure is taken again and your need for the drug can be reassessed.

b) How many times a day the drug should be taken. If a drug needs to be taken once a day it is important that it is taken at the same time each day. If a drug has to be taken twice a day then it should be taken at intervals of twelve hours. A drug that needs to be taken three times a day should be taken at eight hourly intervals (unless you are instructed otherwise) and a drug that needs taking four times a day should usually be taken at six hourly intervals. Modern drugs are powerful and sophisticated; they need to be taken at exactly the right time if the right effects are to be obtained.

c) Whether the drug should be taken before meals, during meals or after meals. Some drugs may cause stomach problems if taken on an empty stomach - they will obviously be safer if taken with food. Other drugs are not properly absorbed if taken with food.

2. When you have been given instructions about how to take a drug follow those instructions carefully.

3. Remember that many drugs do not mix well with alcohol. It is always safer to assume that you should not drink alcohol while taking a drug until you have checked with your doctor.

4. You must not take non-prescribed medicines while taking prescribed medicines unless your doctor has given his approval. The effect of some drugs for the treatment of high blood pressure can be distorted by over-the-counter remedies.

5. Occasionally, drugs do not mix with food. If your doctor tells you not to eat a particular type of food then it is important that you follow his instructions.

6. Keep drugs in a locked cupboard where the temperature is stable. Blood pressure drugs, if taken by children, can be extremely dangerous. Although most of us keep our medicines in the bathroom that is not the best place for them - the temperature and humidity levels there tend to vary too much. Your bedroom is probably best.

7. Do not remove drugs from their proper containers except when you are taking them or when you are transferring them to a special 'day' box to carry around with you.

8. Some drugs prescribed for high blood pressure can cause drowsiness. If you have to drive a motor car or handle any machinery then it is important that you ask your doctor if the drugs he has prescribed will have this side effect.

9. Never, ever take drugs that have been prescribed for someone else. Even if they seem to have the same symptoms as you, even if they have a high blood pressure problem, their pills may not suit you.

10.   It is important that once you start receiving treatment you always try to see the same doctor. One reason for this is that if several doctors are prescribing for you the chances are that your drug regime will become complicated and confusing. Different doctors prefer different drugs for the treatment of high blood pressure. The other important reason for sticking to one doctor is that different doctors measure blood pressure in slightly different ways. If one doctor is a little deafer than another, for example, he may hear the appropriate sounds a few seconds later - and record a different reading. Also, sphygmomanometers can vary.

11.   Be on the look out for side effects and do remember that if you seem to develop a second illness then the chances are high that it is caused by the treatment you are receiving.

12.   Remember, that although drugs need to be used with care and caution they may help save your life. If you need drugs to bring your blood pressure down to normal levels then you must keep taking your drugs. The risks associated with the drugs you are taking are unlikely to be as high as the risks that you would run if your blood pressure was allowed to remain high and uncontrolled.

Side effects

At least forty per cent of the people who take prescribed drugs suffer some form of side effect. Most of the side effects appear within the first four days of treatment. Some are minor and short-lasting; others are permanent, debilitating and dangerous.
       The side effects suffered by patients taking drugs for the treatment of high blood pressure will obviously vary according to the

individual patient and the nature of the drug prescribed. Patients should always be aware of the possibility of side effects developing and should be prepared to report new signs or symptoms to their doctors straight away so that they can decide what to do.

Although all drugs can cause a whole range of side effects, here are some of the side effects which are particularly common with drugs used to control high blood pressure:

- Drowsiness
- Dry mouth
- Impotence
- Loss of interest in sex
- Tiredness
- Hallucinations
- Confusion
- Hypotension
- Breathlessness

If you suffer regularly from one particular type of side effects then your doctor may be able to solve the problem by switching to another type of drug.

The dangers of mixing drugs

If you are prescribed a drug you should never take any other drug unless it has been prescribed for you by a doctor who knows what you are already taking.

Blood pressure drugs tend to be rather sensitive to other chemicals and mixing drugs can be dangerous.

Drugs during pregnancy and breast feeding

If you are pregnant or planning to become pregnant or if you are breast feeding a baby you must tell your doctor. Some of the drugs used to control high blood pressure could damage your baby.

Making drug taking easier

If you need to take more than three tablets a day or if you need to break any of your tablets in half then you should ask your doctor if there are any possible alternatives. The more tablets you have to take the more likely you are to forget a dose - and the less effective your treatment will be. If you have to spend time breaking tablets into halves or quarters then your dosages will become rather irregular as it is difficult to break tablets into equal portions.

There are so many blood pressure control drugs available on the market that your doctor will probably be able to find a product which will help you avoid spending the day swallowing pills or dissecting them on the kitchen table.

Taking drugs on time

It is important that drugs prescribed for the control of high blood pressure are taken on time.

If your doctor has prescribed drugs that need to be taken just once a day then remembering your pills should not be too difficult. If, however, he has given you drugs that need to be taken three times a day, or has give you two or more different types of pills and told you to take one lot twice a day and another lot four times a day then you may have problems.

You can help yourself keep track of your pill taking by making a small daily pill chart. The chart that follows is designed for a patient told to take tablet 1, three times a day; tablet 2, once a day and tablet 3, twice a day.

A fresh chart could be made out for each new day and the individual pills ticked off as they are taken.

	8.00am	4.00pm	8.00pm	Midnight
Tablet 1	1	1	_	1
Tablet 2	1	_	_	_
Tablet 3	1	_	1	_

Going abroad

If you are going out of the country then do remember to take a supply of your pills with you. Some of the products used to control blood pressure are not available internationally and you may find difficulty in obtaining the pills that you have found most effective.

Do remember, too, to keep your pills with you and not to leave them in your luggage. Your blood pressure will not be helped if you end up in Tahiti while your pills are sitting locked in a luggage hold in Hong Kong.

And remember, also, that in hot climates your need for blood pressure pills may be reduced. If you are planning to go somewhere hot you should tell your doctor who may, for example, be able to give you lower dose pills. Alternatively, he can tell you how to reduce your usual medication.

The hazard of hypotension

Occasionally, drugs used to bring down the blood pressure work a little too well - and they reduce the blood pressure too much, producing a condition known as hypotension.

Patients with hypotension usually notice that they feel dizzy or light-headed. These symptoms are worse on sudden movement, as when rising out of a chair or getting up out of bed in the morning. The dizziness usually wears off after a few seconds.

The problem of hypotension is more likely to occur during the hotter weather. Then the body tries to lose heat by pushing as much blood as possible into the blood vessels of the skin. Heat is then lost from the blood and the body manages to keep its internal temperature stable. When the peripheral blood vessels are dilated the existing blood pressure must fall.

If you suffer from dizziness you should visit your doctor as soon as possible so that he can check your blood pressure and, if necessary, adjust your medication. If your hypotension only occurs when it hot then it may simply be enough to reduce your pills during those spells.

Is high blood pressure a permanent problem?

Patients with high blood pressure used to be told that they would need to stay on drugs for ever. I have spoken to a number of patients over the years who have been threatened with all sorts of horrible consequences if they ever dared consider coming off their tablets. 'If you stop taking your pills you will have a stroke,' is a common enough comment from doctors brought up to believe that the only way to deal with high blood pressure is by taking pills.

Although we still do not know exactly what causes high blood pressure we do know that there are a number of specific factors which are often responsible for the development of high blood pressure. (I have already described some of the commonest factors earlier in this book).

And we also know that if these factors are controlled then the blood pressure can often be reduced to normal levels again with the result that it may be possible to stop taking drugs.

So high blood pressure need not be a permanent problem.

Nor do I think that patients with high blood pressure need resign themselves either to taking drugs for the rest of their lives or else dying early from a stroke or a heart attack.

Having said that, do not stop taking your drugs if you have been prescribed them. Before trying to reduce your own blood pressure to safer levels you must first ask your doctor's advice. While changing your lifestyle have your blood pressure checked regularly so that your medication can be adjusted. If and when your blood pressure pills need to be reduced then they must be reduced by your doctor and he must do so while keeping a close eye on your blood pressure.

PART THREE

Blood Pressure Control Programme

Introduction

There is much that you can do to help yourself if your suffer from high blood pressure. There is a very real chance that if you follow the advice in this blood pressure control programme you will be able to control your blood pressure without drugs.

Before starting this programme you must, of course, consult your doctor. As your blood pressure is reduced your need for drugs may change.

Adapt your personality

Earlier, I explained how your personality can affect your chances of developing high blood pressure. There are many other factors which decide whether or not you are going to develop high blood pressure but 'personality' is undoubtedly a critical one. And even though I do not pretend for an instant that you can change your personality (nor do I think that it would be a good idea to try) you can certainly adapt it and your way of life in such a way that your blood pressure will benefit.

a) Deal with aggression and competitiveness

In order to cope with your ambitions you must first decide what your priorities are; and decide which parts of your life are most important. If you let your ambitions spill over into every aspect of your life then you will soon burn yourself out. So, for example, if your job is extremely important to you it is important that you are able to relax when you are playing games. If you take everything seriously you will be pushing yourself too hard - and your blood pressure will rise.

And remember too that however important your ambitions are you will be much more likely to succeed if you are prepared to take time off occasionally to relax. Read the section in this book which deals with mental forms of relaxation. If you are an aggressive, ambitious individual then it is important that you read this part of the book carefully. In addition to spending some time each day relaxing you would probably be wise to out time aside from more complete relaxation. So, for example, make sure that you have a half day every week when you do something that really does not matter too much. And when you are planning to go on holiday try not to get carried away and give yourself too many things to do.

Finally, do learn to recognise the signs which tell you that you are pushing yourself too hard. There may not be any symptoms to show just what is happening to your blood pressure but look out for other symptoms that show that you are making too many demands of your mind and body.

Look, for example, for signs such as indigestion, headaches, nausea, sleeplessness, and tiredness. Those can all be signs that you are putting yourself under too much pressure. If you can get one it might be wise to buy a machine to measure your own blood pressure. You will then be able to see what happens to your blood pressure under different circumstances. That should give you a good idea of just what you can manage without damaging your health.

b) Avoid frustration

Many of the problems that produce frustration can be avoided by a little advance planning. When you are organising something complicated (such as a house move or an important dinner party) make a list of all the things that have to be done. And then go through your list carefully, looking for possible areas where things can go wrong. Then try to ensure that you have prepared contingency plans for dealing with these potential problems.

Do not allow yourself to become too dependent on others, either. These days we all have to be dependent on many other people - and strikes or failures of supplies can easily lead to frustration. If a power dispute is starting then make sure that you have alternative forms of heating and lighting around. If your business depends on one particular product try to make sure that you have an alternative supplier available.

If you have an important appointment to keep make plans to travel early and do something else in the time that may (all being well) be spent waiting.

None of this advice means changing your personality, of course. All it involves is adapting the way you live to ensure that you suffer as little frustration as possible. That is bound to have a beneficial effect on your blood pressure.

c) Control your temper

If you are the sort of individual who gets easily aroused then you should probably learn to get rid of your aggressions in as harmless a way as possible. It is not sensible to try to repress your natural aggressions but neither is it particularly sensible to let your aggression out when you are working or socialising - you are likely to annoy people, make enemies and store up extra stresses and strains for yourself.

There are plenty of harmless ways by which you can rid yourself of aggressive feelings. If your doctor approves take up an active sport, for example, and get rid of your aggressions by slamming a squash ball around or by hammering a tennis ball. Or take up gardening and go and do a little digging when you feel like shouting. Or buy yourself a punch-bag, paint a face on it and pummel that the next time you want to shout or scream at someone. (Some factories and offices have 'angry' rooms these days where workers can get rid of their aggressions.)

Do remember, however, that if you suffer from high blood pressure you should not do anything too physically exhausting!

d) Let your emotions show

Do not store up tears inside you. There is now evidence to show that when we cry there are very good reasons for it: not only does our crying make it clear to those around us that we need extra comfort and attention but the tears we shed contain harmful substances that our body needs to get rid of when we are upset. The research work in this area is still in its infancy but it does seem possible that if you refuse to cry your body will store up harmful chemicals and you will end up with a genuine, full blown depression.

I am not suggesting that you open the floodgates at every possible opportunity. But do not be afraid to cry in front of those who are close to you, or in private. Store up the tears and you will probably make your blood pressure go up.

e) Control your feelings of guilt

First of all you must, of course, decide whether or not any particular feeling of guilt is really justified or not. Obviously, if you are feeling guilty because of something that you have done (run into a parked car or broken a cup, for example) then the only solution is to apologise and make what amends you can. In most instances, however, guilt is far more complex than that. If you are the sort of individual who tends to suffer from guilt then you probably feel guilty for things you have not done and because of your own suspicions about how other people will feel and respond.

This is the type of guilt that causes most pain and to deal with it you must first of all find out exactly why it is you feel guilty. Is it because you feel you have failed someone such as your mother, your employer, your spouse or your god? Much of the guilt we suffer is produced by our relationships with those who are very close to us (love is the greatest single cause of guilt) and so in order to protect yourself more effectively you must learn to differentiate between the realistic expectations of those who are close to you and their unrealistic demands. You must learn not to allow other people to put unreasonable demands on you or your conscience.

So, for example, you should perhaps not feel guilty if you cannot visit your parents every week, if you cannot buy your children all the toys they want, if you cannot do all the overtime that your employer would like you to do - and so on.

The truth about individuals who suffer a lot from guilt is that they tend to be thoughtful and caring people.

If you suffer a lot from pangs of guilt it is probably because you care too much about other people; you probably worry too much about what other people want; about what other people feel and about how your actions are going to be seen by others.

I know that this may sound strange, but to protect yourself a little and to keep your blood pressure under control you need to be a little more selfish, a little more self-aware and a little more able to appreciate your own good points. If you are the sort of person who is driven by guilt then you are probably conscientious, hard working, ambitious, thoughtful, reliable, honest and generous. Despite all these good points you probably think of yourself as a failure and you are probably far too critical about what you do. You probably expect far more from yourself then you would ever dream of expecting from anyone else - and some of the people around you may well take advantage of this trait.

I suggest that you sit yourself down and write out a list of your good points. Pretend that you are writing your own obituary and be honest and fair to yourself. You will almost certainly end up with a fairly long list of good things that you could say about yourself.

Next time you are swamped with guilt look at your list, take a little pride in yourself and learn to be a little more selfish.

f) Deal with worry and anxiety

Fears can be debilitating - and have a bad effect on your blood pressure. To cope with your fears you must recognise and face those things that worry you most. The unknown, unidentified fear is much more dangerous and more damaging than the fear that has been carefully examined.

Once you have made a list of all the things that really worry you, you can go through that list and see what you can do to help yourself worry less. So, for example, if you worry a good deal about your health it might be wise to visit your doctor for a complete check up. Or, better still, make a positive decision to learn more about your body and to come to terms with just what you need to do in order to conquer your problems. Self awareness and understanding will last much longer in your battle against fear than professional reassurance.

If your fears concern money, employment or whatever, the same is true. Once you have made a precise list of all the things that worry you then you are more likely to do something to help yourself. You will not be able to solve all your fears or eradicate all your worries straight away, of course. But you will be able to do something to help yourself. And that always makes a tremendous difference to the way your body and your blood pressure respond.

Learn to relax your body

When you are anxious, nervous or under stress in any way your mind deliberately tenses up the muscles around your body. There is a long established, sensible reason for this. By tensing up muscles your mind is preparing your body for action; it assumes that the best way to deal with the threat you are facing will be physical action. Your mind is getting your body ready to fight or to run away.

But most modern stresses cannot be dealt with by a physical response. You cannot fight a traffic jam and running away from an electricity bill won't do you any good. Modern stresses persist for long periods - and so muscles remain tense for long periods too.

Tensed muscles commonly produce headaches, backache and stiff necks. Eight out of ten cases of backache are caused by stress and a staggering 98 per cent of headaches are produced in the same way.

Learning how to avoid unnecessary stresses, how to build up your resistance to stress and how to improve your ability to cope with stress will all help you combat muscle tension.

But there is another, more direct way, to tackle muscle tension and the associated problems it produces: deliberately relaxing your tensed muscles.

Relaxing your body

Make sure that you will not be disturbed for at least twenty minutes then lie down somewhere quiet and comfortable and use this simple-to-learn technique to help relieve muscle tension.

1.   Take very deep, slow breaths. Stress will make you breathe more quickly than usual so soothe your mind - and your body - by deliberately taking slower, deeper breaths.

2.   Clench your left hand as tightly as you can, making a fist with your fingers. Do it well and you will see the knuckles go white. If you now let your fist unfold you will feel the muscles relax. When your hand was clenched the muscles were tensed; unfolded the same muscles are relaxed. This is what you must do with the other muscle groups of your body.

3.   Bend your left arm and try to make your left biceps muscle stand out as much as you can. Then relax it and let the muscles ease. When your arm is thoroughly relaxed let it lie loosely by your side.

4.   Clench your right hand as tightly as you can, making a fist again with your fingers. When you let your fist unfold you will feel the muscles relax.

5.   Now bend your right arm and make your right biceps muscle stand out as much as you can. Then relax it and let the muscles become relaxed. When your arm is thoroughly relaxed let it lie loosely by your side.

6.   Tighten the muscles in your left foot. Curl your toes upwards. And then downwards. When your foot feels as tense as you can make it deliberately relax the muscles.

7. Tense the muscles of your left calf. You should be able to feel the muscles in the back of your left leg become firm and hard as you tense them. Bend your foot up towards you to help tighten the muscles. Then let the muscles relax.

8. Straighten your left leg and point your foot away from you. You will feel the muscles on the front of your left thigh tighten up - they should be firm right up to the top of your leg. Now relax those muscles and let your left leg lie loosely on the bed.

9. Tighten the muscles in your right foot. Curl your toes upwards. And then downwards. When your foot feels as tense as you can make it deliberately relax the muscles.

10. Tense the muscles of your right calf. You should be able to feel the muscles in the back of your right leg become firm and hard as you tense them. Bend your foot up towards you to help tighten the muscles. Then let the muscles relax.

11. Straighten your right leg and point your foot away from you. You will feel the muscles on the front of your right thigh tighten up - they should be firm right up to the top of your leg. Now relax those muscles and let your right leg lie loosely on the bed.

12. Lift yourself up by tightening your buttock muscles. You should be able to lift your body upwards by an inch or so. Then let your muscles fall loose again.

13. Tense and contract your abdominal muscles. Try to pull your abdominal wall as far in as possible. Then let go and allow your waist to reach its maximum circumference.

14. Tighten up the muscles of your chest. Take a big, deep breath in and hold it for as long as possible. Then, slowly, let it go.

15. Push your shoulders backwards as far as they will go, then bring them forwards and inwards. Finally, shrug them as high as you can. Keep your head perfectly still and try to touch your ears with your shoulders. It will probably be impossible but try anyway. Then let your shoulders relax and ease.

16.   Next tighten up the muscles of your back. Try to make yourself as tall as you can. Then let the muscles relax.

17.   The muscles of your neck are next. Lift your head forwards and turn your head first one way and then the other. Then let the muscles of your neck relax. Move your head around and make sure that your neck muscles are completely loose and easy.

18.   Move your eyebrows upwards and then pull them down as far as they will go. Do this several times, making sure that you can feel the muscles tightening both when you move your eyebrows up and when you pull them down. Then let them relax.

19.   Screw up your eyes as tightly as you can. Pretend that someone is trying to force your eyes open. Keep them shut tightly. Then, keeping your eyelids closed, let them relax.

20.   Move your lower jaw around. Grit your teeth. Wrinkle your nose. Smile as wide as you can showing as many teeth as you can. Push your tongue out as far as it will go, push it firmly against the bottom of your mouth and then the top of your mouth before letting it lie easy and relaxed inside your mouth. Now let all your facial muscles go loose and relaxed.

Make your own relaxation tape

To make your own relaxation tape slowly read out the 'Relaxing Your Body' script into a tape recorder. Then lie down, play back the tape and listen to it carefully. You'll find it much easier to listen to the instructions on a tape than to try and read them out of a book while you are relaxing. Do remember to read out the instructions fairly slowly - and to pause between each set of instructions. You may need one or two attempts to get it absolutely right.

Too busy to relax?

Busy people often say that they are too busy to relax. They say that relaxing is a waste of time.

They're wrong!

Learning to relax is as essential for your mind as eating is for your body.

Learn to relax your mind

One of the easiest and most effective ways to deal with stress and to stop anxiety, fear and worry affecting your blood pressure is to learn how to relax your mind. There is now evidence from all parts of the world to show that patients with high blood pressure have learned to control their pressure simply by learning how to relax their minds - many, many patients have been able to stop taking drugs simply by using mind relaxing techniques.

Under normal, everyday circumstances an unending stream of facts and feelings pours into your mind. Even when you are not consciously 'thinking', your eyes, ears, nose and other sense organs will be pushing thousands of bits and pieces of unwanted information into your mind. Together, all these pieces of information help to produce stress and pressure. If you can cut out the number of messages going into your brain then you will be able to ease the amount of pressure on your mind. And the effect on your blood pressure will almost certainly be beneficial.

Many of the people who recommend mental relaxation suggest that you should try to empty your mind completely in order to cut out the damaging effect of all this information.

The problem is, of course, that trying to empty your mind of all the conscious and subconscious messages that keep streaming into it is not easy. Indeed, very many people find the prospect of emptying their minds completely so terrifying that they never even try. And so they lose the possibility of benefiting from simple mental relaxation.

Fortunately, however, there is another way to cut down the amount of damaging information pouring into your mind. And that is to fill your mind with pleasant, peaceful, relaxing thoughts. In other words, all you have to do is re-learn how to daydream. I say re-learn deliberately because you will almost certainly have been able to daydream when you were small. But you were probably taught (by both your parents and your teachers) that daydreaming is wasteful and rather naughty.

Daydreaming works for several reasons. First, it works because your body will respond to an imagined world just as effectively as it will respond to the real world. When the film 'Lawrence of Arabia' was first shown cinema managers around the world were astonished to find that the sales of cold drinks and ice creams rocketed. Even when the heating failed in one particular cinema and the temperature plummeted the patrons still wanted to buy cold drinks and ice creams. The explanation was that the cinema patrons were responding to the desert scenes that they were watching on the screen. Their bodies responded as though the desert was entirely real. So, fill your mind with some pleasant, relaxing, imaginary scene and your body will respond as though the scene were real. The horrors of the real world around you will be forgotten.

The second reason why daydreaming works so well is that the human body responds positively to good, happy, feelings. When we are frightened or worried we respond badly: our blood pressure goes up, we feel upset, we get indigestion and so on. But when we are happy and contented there is a very clear and useful healing effect on the body. So, if you learn how to daydream you will benefit in both those ways. And your blood pressure will very probably come down.

When you begin re-learning how to daydream you will probably have to find yourself somewhere quiet and peaceful. You will need to be able to cut out the world. Later on, when you have mastered the art, you will be able to do it just about anywhere.

So, to start with, lie yourself down on your bed, close the door, take the telephone off the hook, feed the animals and draw the curtains. Put a 'Do Not Disturb' notice on the door.

Once you are peacefully settled try to remember some particularly happy and peaceful scene from your past. It is best to use a
real scene because you will be better able to re-create all the necessary feelings. But you can, if you like, use an entirely fictional scene.

If you are using a scene from your past then you might try a
beach scene from a good holiday by the sea. With your eyes firmly
closed take big, deep breaths as slowly and as regularly as you
possibly can. And then slowly try to feel the warmth of the sun on
your face. Try not to let anyone else into your daydream by the way.
If you let people into your daydream then you are likely to either
end up with a nightmare or with a fantasy. And neither is likely to be
particularly relaxing.

Once you can feel the sun on your face try to imagine that you
can hear the sound of the waves breaking on the shore. And try too
to feel the warm, soft sand underneath you. Listen to the seagulls
circling overhead and smell the salty sea air. Allow a gentle breeze
to play over your body.

Once your mind has been convinced your body will be convinced too. The accumulated pressures from the real world will
slowly disappear. As your mind is filled with all these peaceful
thoughts so your body will begin to respond. Your blood pressure
will begin to fall.

You do not, of course, have to restrict yourself to this one
particular daydream. You can build up your very own, personal
library of useful daydreams. There can be real memories, there can
be fictional memories and there can be memories taken from films
or books. It does not matter what the memory is as long as the
effect is to make you feel happy and peaceful, and as long as you
can create memories that are convincing.

Reduce your stress by organising your life

The motorist who remembers to buy petrol for his car will be far
less likely to find himself stressed by running out of fuel on the mo-

torway. The shopper who knows in advance what he is going to buy will be far less likely to end up making a second trip to the shops. The businessman who plans ahead will be far less likely to end up with a 'crisis' on his hands. Bad organisation and poor planning often lead to anxiety, to increased stress loads and to high blood pressure. Learn to organise your life and you will reduce the number of crises which might make your blood pressure go up.
Follow this simple four-stage plan.

1. Keep a diary that contains details of all events that need advance planning (birthdays, anniversaries etc). Get into the habit of examining it each morning to make sure that you know just what you have to do. Advance planning for trips and meetings of all kinds obviously helps to reduce the risk of something going wrong.

2. Keep an efficient filing system to enable you to store bills, letters and receipts just where you can find them. There is nothing more frustrating (and worse for your blood pressure) than hunting around for an important letter and wasting hours on the job. You do not have to buy a filing cabinet - you can use old brown envelopes or a cardboard box.

3. When you have a really difficult problem to solve do not let it ruin your life - simply write down all the possible solutions in a notebook. Keep the list somewhere safe and near to you and add new solutions as they occur to you. Keep the list by you when you are in the bath, in the car or in bed: those are the places where ideas tend to come to you. Then, when you finally need to make a decision take a look down your list of possibilities and you will probably find that one particular answer stands out. You will certainly be able to cross out many of the alternatives which seemed logical when you wrote them down but which now look silly.

4. Keep a notebook and a pencil with you at all times. Jot down any thought that needs remembering or needs action. When they are put down on paper, problems always seem slightly less significant. And you will not have to worry about remembering them either.

Control your weight

Losing weight can make a dramatic difference to blood pressure. Indeed, it is one of the most effective ways to reduce it.

There are two ways of losing excess weight.

The first is to increase the amount of work and exercise that you do while keeping your food intake fairly stable. You need to increase your daily exercise regime fairly substantially, however, in order to burn up food faster than you are taking it into your body. This is, I know, the solution that many people favour these days and a large number of the joggers who set out each morning in their track suits and woolly hats hope to lose weight. Unfortunately, exercising is not a practical or particularly effective way of losing weight. The sad truth is that to lose weight by exercising you have virtually to become a professional athlete, forever running, lifting and working out. A little, occasional, mild exercise just will not make any real difference.

The second solution is to reduce your food intake so that it falls below your body's requirements. Do this and your body will need to take food from your stored supplies - and you will lose weight.

The problem with this sensible, sound and efficient solution is, of course, that eating less than you need can be difficult and even painful.

Before I explain how I think you can manage to lose weight relatively painlessly and easily I want to discuss the other major problem that all dieters have to face - keeping the food intake down afterwards so that the excess weight does not come back straight away. Losing weight is, like giving up smoking, very easy: hundreds of thousands of people do it many times a year. The difficult part is staying slim.

The reason why I want to discuss this problem now is that if you understand why you are likely to put weight back on again after dieting then you will not only understand the sort of things which make your dieting fail but you will also understand what you need to do to lose weight without too much pain or discomfort.

Anyone wanting to lose weight should know that there is an appetite control centre in the human brain which is designed to ensure that you eat exactly what your body needs and in precisely the quantities that are needed.

This appetite control centre is so sophisticated that it can change your diet if your circumstances change. So, for example, research done with soldiers has shown that when men are suddenly put down in the desert or in the Arctic wastes they will unconsciously change their dietary habits to fit in with their circumstances. Their bodies' needs vary according to the environment and the appetite control centre makes the appropriate signals to adjust dietary habits.

The reason why so many of us get fat is that we eat the wrong foods, at the wrong times and in the wrong amounts. And we do this because we eat for all the wrong reasons. We eat food that looks good; we eat foods that have been promoted on television; we eat up everything on our plates whether or not we are hungry simply because when we were small we were told by our mothers that we should never leave food to go to waste; we eat at fixed meal times that are often decided by other people; we eat because other people are eating and we want to look sociable; we eat because we are upset and we have always associated food with feeling good and so on and so on.

In other words we no longer listen to our appetite control centres; we eat for all the wrong reasons.

And this explains not only why so many of us are overweight, but why we so often find it difficult to keep weight off once we have dieted successfully. As soon as we have finished dieting we simply go back to our old, bad habits and we put all the weight back on again.

If you are going to lose your excess weight and keep it off then you have to get back into the habit of eating according to your body's needs and not eating according to other people's wishes. You have to learn to listen to your body's internal signs of hunger, learn to break bad eating habits, and learn to eat the foods you need, when you need them and in the quantities you need.

To maintain your weight you need to follow these rules:

1. You must concentrate on what you are doing when you are eating. If you are reading, talking or watching television while you are eating you will miss the all-important messages from your appetite control centre.

2. You must make absolutely sure that you only ever eat when you are hungry. Every time a piece of food is on its way to your mouth you must ask yourself whether or not you are genuinely hungry. If you are hungry - then eat it. If you are not really hungry but you are eating for some other reason then stop.

3. Never, ever be frightened to leave food on the side of your plate if you have had more than you need. I know it is a waste to throw food away but its just as much a waste (and likely to do your body untold damage) to eat it. This is something that most of us find difficult to do - largely because we were taught as children that it is sinful to waste food. Fortunately, when you find that you are having to leave food on the side of your plate you can easily solve the problem for the future by serving yourself smaller portions.

4. You are better off eating small meals regularly than huge meals every now and then. If you eat occasionally your body will store up excess food because it will know that it might be some time before more food comes its way. If you eat small meals fairly regularly, the food will be burnt up quite quickly. Nibbling is better for you than stuffing yourself at meal times.

5. Do make sure that you never use food as a crutch. Do not promise yourself food as a prize or a reward. Do not eat to cheer yourself up. It is an easy habit to form but a difficult one to break.

Following these simple instructions will take a little effort to start with. If you have spent years of your life acquiring bad eating habits it will take longer to get into the habit of eating sensibly.

The reward, though, is that your weight will remain stable. And, hopefully, your blood pressure will remain under control.

To lose weight

If you want to lose weight then you have somehow to trick your appetite control centre into thinking that you have put enough food into your body. You must convince yourself that you are no longer hungry, even though you have eaten less food than your body needs. If you can do this then your body will draw on stored fat supplies and you will lose weight.

There are several simple tricks that you can try.

When you feel hungry eat filling but low-calorie snacks. Drink a glass of one-calorie squash or cola; or a cup of black coffee or lemon tea; or a bowl of clear soup. You will feel full without having filled your body with calories.

Another trick is to have a small snack half an hour before a main meal. A piece of raw fruit, or a hunk of vegetable will do. The aim is to spoil your appetite, convince your body that you are no longer hungry and stop you eating as much as you really need.

You can also help yourself by picking foods that take a lot of chewing (foods such as raw vegetables). This will slow you down and make you more aware of when you have eaten enough.

Become a vegetarian

The evidence suggests that vegetarians tend to have lower blood pressure than people who eat meat. And if you have high blood pressure then starting on a vegetarian diet could help bring your blood pressure down. This could be because meat contains a lot of sodium. But it could also be because meat often contains a lot of fat. I don't think anyone yet knows precisely why a vegetarian diet is better for high blood pressure sufferers - but I certainly believe that it is.

Avoid dairy produce

Although some types of milk and cheese contain less fat than others a diet which contains a good deal of diary produce will usually contain a good deal of fat. I suggest that high blood pressure sufferers should reduce their intake of butter, cheese, milk and cream.

Reduce your salt intake

The evidence now available suggests that anyone who has high blood pressure should make an attempt to reduce his salt intake. This is best done be avoiding the following foods (or, at least, keeping their consumption down to a minimum):

> *processed foods in general*
> *canned foods*
> *junk foods (such as take away hamburgers etc)*
> *crisps*
> *salted peanuts*
> *cheese crackers*
> *chips*
> *lobsters*
> *oysters*
> *salted butter and cheese*

sausages
bacon
milk and milk products

You should also avoid adding salt when cooking food. And salt should be banished from the table.

If you find saltless food unappetising there are a number of other flavourings that you can try.

These include:
lemon juice
parsley
garlic
horseradish
tarragon

Increase your potassium intake

Just as there is evidence to show that too much salt has an adverse effect on patients with high blood pressure so there is also evidence to show that some patients with blood pressure problems are deficient in potassium. Increase your consumption of foods that are rich in potassium.

These include:
apples
apricots
asparagus
avocados
bananas
beans
brussels sprouts
cauliflower

corn on the cob
dates
grapefruit juice
lentils
orange juice
peach
peas
pineapple juice
prunes
potatoes (though not as fatty, salted chips!)
rhubarb
spinach
sunflower seeds
tomato juice

Reduce your intake of animal fats

Animal fats can kill and you need to keep your intake of such products to a minimum. You should eat less:

meat (ideally you should follow a vegetarian diet)
eggs
butter
milk
cream

You should also grill rather than fry your food when possible. And you should cook with vegetable oils.

Reduce your caffeine intake

Caffeine shrinks blood vessels and has an adverse effect on blood pressure levels. I do not think there is any need to cut out caffeine completely but if you are drinking more than three or four cups of strong coffee or tea each day or you drink many cola drinks then you should try to cut down.

Control your intake of alcohol

You should not drink more than two or three glasses of alcohol (beer, wine, spirits) in any one day. If you drink less than this on one day do not transfer that 'allocation' to another day.

Stop smoking

Any method you choose that works is a good one! Some people claim that they have managed to give up smoking by visiting a hypnotist; others that special chewing gum helped them more than anything else. I once came across a man who managed by eating prunes. Heaven know what sort of effect that had on his bowels but it apparently helped him 'kick' the tobacco habit.

Before you try to give up find out exactly why you smoke. If you do it to help you relieve your stress then giving it up without doing anything else to help you cope with stress may result in an increase in your blood pressure - rather than a decrease. If you usually inhale when you are smoking then you are very probably addicted to tobacco, and, for you, giving up smoking is likely to be a physical strain. If you rarely smoke by yourself but merely smoke when you are with friends then your habit is probably a social one.

Once you have decided just why you smoke - and you have done what you can to ensure that giving up smoking is not likely to have a damaging effect on your life - then you can set up the practical business of giving up tobacco.

The techniques described below are ones that have been found to work:

1.   If you have an economical mind then you will probably find that it helps to write down each day just how much money you have

saved (or would have saved) by not smoking. It adds up quickly and by the end of a month the amount may be substantial.

2. If you usually smoke one particular type of cigarette try changing the brand you buy every time you buy a new pack. This will make life rather difficult because you will be constantly looking for new brands. It will also make smoking a less familiar occupation. Some cigarettes will be weaker: others stronger. Buy them from a different shop, too. Never buy more than one pack at once; buy in packs of ten; and try to remember to forget to take your cigarettes with you when you go out.

3. Make a list of all the places where you smoke. Put every single place on your list - bedroom, car, restaurant, office, bus, train, lavatory, lifts, streets, shops, friends homes, bathroom, garden, pub, telephone kiosks etc. Then write out the places again, this time with the places where you do least smoking at the bottom, and the places where you do most at the top.

Now, stop smoking in each place in turn, starting with the one that is at the bottom. So, for example, if it is the garden make sure that you do not smoke there on day one. Put a tick by 'garden' to remind you just how far you have got. Then, on day two, do not smoke in the place that is next to the bottom. If, for example it is the bathroom make sure that you do not smoke there.

And carry on, day by day, working your way up the list. You must remember, of course, that as you go up the list you cannot smoke anywhere that you have already ticked. So, on day three, for example, you cannot smoke in the garden or the bathroom or in the place that is third up the list.

The main advantage with this system is that it will enable you to give up smoking at an acceptable rate. Even if you do not manage to give up smoking altogether you will have managed to give up a bit - and that will help. The other advantage is that it allows you to carry on smoking in those places where you need to smoke most of all. So, if your office is right at the top of your list and that is where you are under most stress and most likely to need the comfort of a cigarette you will be able to smoke there right until the end.

Remember, too, as you give up smoking that even if you can only cut down (rather than give up altogether) that will have a noticeable effect on your health and will reduce the risk of your blood pressure giving you major problems in the future.

Take up gentle exercise

A good deal of nonsense has been talked about exercise in recent years. Everywhere you turn there are actresses, singers and celebrities insisting that they have a secret exercise solution to good health. The leotard business has never been better and there are hundreds of pushy entrepreneurs selling rowing machines, weight lifting contraptions, track suits, running shoes and all sorts of other gadgets.

The claims that have been made by all these 'experts' have made exercise sound like a universal panacea. Whether they are encouraging you to take up aerobic exercise, gymnastics, weight lifting or squash, the experts will insist that their sport will help you live longer, stay fitter and avoid problems like high blood pressure.

I am afraid that a good deal of this talk has been based not on sound clinical and scientific principles but on commercially inspired rhetoric. The truth is that too much exercise will damage and weaken your body.

There are two main problems with the sort of exercise that is recommended by the exercise enthusiasts.

First, they sometimes seem to insist that it is vital to go through the pain barrier in order to benefit from an exercise programme. I contend that it is positively dangerous to try and go through a real pain barrier and that people who insist on following this sort of foolhardy advice will end up injuring themselves. Pain is one of the body's natural defence mechanisms. When we exercise and we get a pain the pain is there for a purpose - it is designed to make us stop what we are doing.

The exercise freaks argue that if you continue to exercise you can force your way through to the pain barrier.

I agree with them on this point but the fact is that when anyone goes through the pain barrier the body produces its own pain relieving hormones simply because it is under the impression that a major crisis requires the body to keep moving. If a soldier hurts his ankle while running across a battle field his first reaction will be to stop and rest his ankle for a while. If, however, he is being chased by enemy soldiers he will want to get up and carry on running. His body, recognising that the need to keep running over-rides the need to protect damaged ankle, will produce internal pain relieving hormones. The pain of the injured ankle will be temporarily forgotten.

This is why marathon runners can keep going when they have injured themselves. The problem is, of course, that by continuing to run on the injured joint the runner is damaging the joint. He may end up with a serious injury that will require long-term, professional treatment. (The injured soldier running away to save his life would probably damage his joint too but he would probably be quite happy to accept such a small price in return for his life). This is why approximately one third of all joggers and runners need specialist orthopaedic or osteopathic treatment every year.

The second reason why the exercise enthusiasts often do more harm than good is that they invariably take themselves far too seriously. Many of the people who take up exercise to get fit become quite dedicated to their sport. They become anxious to do well and they put themselves under stress to run faster, lift more weights, or beat another player at tennis, badminton or squash.

Anyone who has high blood pressure will probably be under enough stress from other areas in their life without adding more from this source.

Having said that, gentle, regular exercise, taken for fun and enjoyed as a form of relaxation, will help anyone suffering from high blood pressure.

There is not, I am afraid, any evidence to show that exercise actually helps reduce blood pressure. But many sufferers have found that gentle exercise does give them a feeling of well being and there are certainly many doctors happy to recommend it.

Just what sort of exercise you choose should depend on your

personal preferences. Cycling, swimming and dancing are three quite excellent, natural types of exercise that many people enjoy. If you are not sure what to try then I suggest walking. Do not set yourself targets or push yourself if you think you have had enough, and do remember that if walking reduces your blood pressure then you may feel a little dizzy and need to rest occasionally. Remember, when you start your modest exercise programme, that if you enjoy your exercise it will undoubtedly reduce your stress levels. So you will benefit twice!

Keep a check on your own blood pressure

Measuring your own blood pressure at home has several advantages:

1. You can take weekly readings which will give you a more accurate picture of your blood pressure than readings taken once every three or six months at a doctor's surgery.

2. Most people's blood pressure rises automatically when they go into a doctor's surgery. Taking your blood pressure at home enables you to avoid this problem.

3. If you take your own blood pressure and keep a chart of your readings you can see how effective your blood pressure control programme is.

4. You can make sure that you always take your blood pressure at the same time of day. (Blood pressures vary from one time of day to another. It tends to be highest at about ten am and lowest at about three am.)

Several types of sphygmomanometer are available for home use. Check yours alongside your doctor's machine.

Wear a medical bracelet or necklace

I suggest that patients who have high blood pressure and/or are regularly treated with drugs wear some sort of identification bracelet, carrying details of their condition and of treatment they are receiving. Some pharmacies sell suitable jewellery. Otherwise ask your doctor for help.

Alternative treatments

I know of no safe and efficient 'over the counter' drugs for the treatment of high blood pressure. Its treatment is one area where orthodox medicine really does have the best - and only - answers. Alternative or complementary forms of medicine are playing an increasingly large part in medical care but there are no alternative forms of treatment that I know of which match the types of treatment offered by orthodox medical practitioners.

However, I have no doubt that there are some alternative remedies which may help people relax, lose weight, give up smoking and make other lifestyle changes which will bring down their blood pressure.

Other books by Vernon Coleman

How To Overcome Toxic Stress
and the Twentieth Century Blues

*'Never have I read a book that is so startlingly true. I was
dumbfounded by your wisdom. You will go down in history as
one of the truly great health reformers of our time'*
(Extracted from a letter to the author)

If you are frustrated, bored, lonely, angry, sad, tired, listless,
frightened, unhappy or tearful then it is possible that you are
suffering from Toxic Stress.
    After two decades of research Dr Coleman has come up
with his own antidote to Toxic Stress which he shares with you
in this inspirational book. In order to feel well and happy again
you need to take a close look at your life and put things back in
the right order. Dr Coleman shows you how to value the worth-
while things in life and give less time to things which matter
very little at all. The book contains hundreds of practical tips on
how to cope with the stresses and strains of daily life.

Price £9.95

Published by European Medical Journal
Order from Publishing House, Trinity Place, Barnstaple,
Devon EX32 9HJ, England

Other books by Vernon Coleman

Food For Thought

Between a third and a half of all cancers may be caused by eating the wrong foods. In this bestselling book Dr Coleman explains which foods to avoid and which to eat to reduce your risk of developing cancer. He also lists foods known to be associated with a wide range of other diseases including Asthma, Gall Bladder Disease, Headaches, Heart Trouble, High Blood Pressure, Indigestion and many more.

Years of research have gone into the writing of this book which explains the facts about mad cow disease, vegetarian eating, microwaves, drinking water, food poisoning, food irradiation and additives. It contains all the information you need about vitamins, carbohydrates, fats and proteins plus a list of 20 superfoods which Dr Coleman believes can improve your health and protect you from a wide range of health problems. The book also includes a "slim-for-life" programme with 48 quick slimming tips to help you lose weight safely and permanently.

" ... a guide to healthy eating which reads like a thriller"
(The Good Book Guide)

"Dr Vernon Coleman is one of our most enlightened, trenchant and sensible dispensers of medical advice"
(The Observer)

Price £9.95

Published by EMJ Books
Order from Publishing House, Trinity Place, Barnstaple,
Devon EX32 9HJ, England

Also available by Vernon Coleman

Betrayal of Trust

Vernon Coleman catalogues the incompetence and dishonesty of the medical profession and the pharmaceutical industry and explains the historical background to the problems which exist today in the world of healthcare. He shows how drugs are put onto the market without being properly tested, and provides hard evidence for his astonishing assertion that doctors do more harm than good.

"I found (it) so brilliant I could not stop reading it"
(A.P., Luton)

"This blast against the medical establishment certainly makes for a rattling good read"
(The Good Book Guide)

"I urge anyone interested in medicine and the safety of drugs to read Betrayal of Trust"
(Leicester Mercury)

"I feel you should be congratulated for producing something that should be required reading for both consumers and producers of the health service"
(R.P., Senior Lecturer in Psychology)

Price £9.95

Published by EMJ Books
Order from Publishing House, Trinity Place, Barnstaple, Devon EX32 9HJ, England

Other books by Vernon Coleman

The Traditional Home Doctor

Vernon Coleman has been writing about health matters for over 25 years and readers have sent him countless thousands of tips and helpful hints. These tips and hints are the sort of information that isn't going to go out of date; they are good, old-fashioned, tried-and-tested methods that have worked for people over the years.

You will find this book a great help the next time you are faced with a family health problem.

The book contains easy-to-follow tips on:

Allergies	Anorexia
Babies	Backache
Burns	Catarrh
Colds	Flu
Constipation	Cystitis
Hay Fever	High Blood Pressure
Headaches	Indigestion
Stress	Prostate Problems
Sleeplessness	Women's Problems
Tiredness	and much more

Each topic includes tips and hints for solving the problem or reducing troublesome symptoms.

Price £9.95

Published by EMJ Books
Order from Publishing House, Trinity Place, Barnstaple, Devon EX32 9HJ, England

Also available by Vernon Coleman

The Bilbury Chronicles

A young doctor arrives to begin work in the small village of Bilbury. This picturesque hamlet is home to some memorable characters who have many a tale to tell, and Vernon Coleman weaves together a superb story full of humour and anecdotes. The Bilbury books will transport you back to the days of old-fashioned, traditional village life where you never needed to lock your door, and when a helping hand was only ever a moment away. The first novel in the series.

"I am just putting pen to paper to say how very much I enjoyed The Bilbury Chronicles. I just can't wait to read the others."
(Mrs K., Cambs)

"...a real delight from cover to cover. As the first in a series it holds out the promise of entertaining things to come"
(Daily Examiner)

"The Bilbury novels are just what I've been looking for. They are a pleasure to read over and over again"
(Mrs C., Lancs)

Price £12.95 (hardback)

Published by Chilton Designs Publishers
Order from Publishing House, Trinity Place, Barnstaple, Devon EX32 9HJ, England

Also available by Vernon Coleman

The Village Cricket Tour

This superb novel tells the story of a team of amateur cricketers who spend two weeks of their summer holidays on tour in
the West Country. It proves to be a most eventful fortnight
full of mishaps and adventures as the cricketers play their
way around the picturesque coastline of Devon and Corn-
wall.

"The only word to describe (this book) is hilarious. It is the
funniest book about cricket that I have ever read. In fact it is the
funniest book I have read since Three Men in a Boat. Anyone
interested in cricket will find this book irresistible."
(Chronicle & Echo)

Price £12.95 (hardback)

Published by Chilton Designs Publishers
Order from Publishing House, Trinity Place, Barnstaple,
Devon EX32 9HJ, England

Telephone 01271 328892
Fax 01271 328768